I0479616

A Healthy Gut Means A Healthy You – A Definitive Guide To Gut Microbiome And Its Benefits

Disclaimer:

This book is not intended as a substitute for the medical advice of physicians. The reader should regularly consult a physician in matters relating to his/her health and particularly concerning any symptoms that may require diagnosis or medical attention.

This book contains general medical information. The medical information is not advice and should not be treated as such.

You must not rely on the information in this book as an alternative to medical advice from your doctor or another professional healthcare provider.

If you have any specific queries about any medical or health condition, you must consult your doctor or a professional healthcare provider.

Based on the information given in this eBook, you should never delay medical attention or disregard medical assistance.

FDA Disclosure

The information in this book has not been evaluated by the Food & Drug Administration or any other medical body. We do not aim to diagnose, treat, cure or prevent any illness or disease. Information is shared for educational purposes only. You must consult your doctor before acting on any content on this website, especially if you are pregnant, nursing, taking medication, or have a medical condition.

Product Link Disclaimer:

I am not getting any endorsement from the companies of the products mentioned in this book. There are no affiliate links and I do not get any affiliate commission if you purchase products through the links present in this book.

Contents

Chapter 1: A Basic Introduction To Probiotics ...1

Introduction 1

A Brief History Of Probiotics 5

Chapter 2: Probiotics Are Real And Scientifically Proven... 7

Do Probiotics Really Help – Exploring The Other Side 8

Researches And Scientific Evidence In Favor Of Probiotics 9

The Different Types Of Probiotics And Their Roles In The Human Body 14

Lactobacillus 15

Lactobacillus Health Benefits To Human Body 16

Bifidobacterium Health Benefits To Human Body 20

Bifidobacterium Longum 22

Chapter 3: The Development Of Probiotics In The Human Body... 23

What Probiotics Mean For Infants And Growing Babies 24

Probiotics And Its Effects On Various Body Systems 27

Probiotics And The Nervous System – The Gut-Brain Axis 28

Probiotics And Cognitive Functions 30

Probiotics And The Metabolism...............32

Probiotics And The Immune System 33

Probiotics And The Respiratory System ...35

Some Diseases That Probiotics May Help Cure 38

- Crohn's Disease................................39

- Irritable Bowel Syndrome (IBS) 41

- Obesity 44

- Diarrhea 46

- Ulcerative Colitis 48

- Vaginal Infections............................49

- Bladder Cancer Recurrence..............51

Chapter 4: Prebiotics Are Not Probiotics 52

What Are Prebiotics? 53

Benefits Of Prebiotics For Human Health 54

- Boost Bacterial Composition Of Hind Gut 55

- Help Reduce Cancer Risk..................55

- Help You Control Blood Pressure.....56

- Improve Nutrient Absorption 56

- Help To Maintain Hormone Health..57

- Improve Immune Functions And Reduces Inflammation 57

- Decrease Risk Of Heart Diseases......58

Best Sources Of Prebiotics 58

- Asparagus...59

- Bananas...59

- Onions...60

- Garlic 60

Best Fermented Foods For Healthy Gut Microbiome 60

Yogurt 61

Kefir..61

Tempeh 62

Chapter 5: The Best Recipes Packed With Gut-healthy Probiotics 63

Kombucha Tea 63

Ingredients 64

Directions..64

Coconut Milk Yogurt 65

Ingredients 65

Directions..66

Almond Milk Kefir 67

Ingredients 68

Directions..68

Kimchi 68

Ingredients 69

Directions..70

Sauerkraut 71

Ingredients 71

Directions..71

Lacto – Fermented Salsa 72

Ingredients 73

Directions..73

Tempeh..73

Directions..75

Miso 75

Ingredients 76

Directions..76

Beet Kvass 76

   Ingredients 77

   Directions 77

Chapter 6: The Role Of Probiotics In The Future
....78

  The Current Stance Of Probiotics In The
  Human Health 78

  Can Probiotics Prove To Be Revolutionary For
  Human Health In The Coming Times?..........80

Conclusion...81

  Appendix 82

  Best Supplements For An Adequate
  Probiotics Supply 82

   BlueBioitics Ultimate Care 82

   Flora Critical Care......................................83

   Garden Of Life Raw Probiotics 83

Chapter 1: A Basic Introduction To Probiotics

Introduction

A holistic healthcare approach aims to empower YOU to take care of yourself and wellbeing. This approach allows you to live life to its fullest and it all starts with you. The power of knowing yourself fuels your lifestyle and helps you find out what works for your body.

The "Gut Health," in this regard, plays a vital role in keeping you happy and healthy. Although the term refers specifically to your intestinal health in the medical domain, the effects are on your overall wellbeing. The gastrointestinal system is a complete digestive process where food enters the mouth, then passes through the esophagus, stomach, small intestine, large intestine, and then passed out of the body via rectum.

Many people think of their gastrointestinal tract as a hollow tube that helps in digestion of the food. Recent scientific discoveries reveal plenty of important functions that your digestion tract performs, such as:

- Changing the brain activation pattern
- Developing the intestinal barrier's functionality and structure
- Developing a significant antibiotic resistance gene when a fetus is in the mother's womb
- Providing the resilience of gut microbiota
- Tuning the immune system to identify between safe and dangerous bacteria

Your GI tract cannot perform all these functions alone and depends on the microbes living in your digestive tract. These microorganisms are yeast and bacteria. In medical terminology, these are the "Gut Microbiota *or Gut Microbiome*" This might sound bizarre, but your gastrointestinal tract contains trillions of microbiota to help it perform the different functions.

The number of microbes that reside within us are more than the cells in your entire body! Over time, our human bodies have developed a complex relationship with these bacteria and microbes that reside within us. Simply put, both you and your microorganism depend on each other to survive. These microbes or probiotics are good bacteria that create the healthy gut microbiome.

That is to say; your gut influences your wellbeing. For instance, if you suffer from nausea, abdominal pain, severe heartburn, or stomach-ache, these symptoms will interfere with your routine and affect your productivity. The impact can be severe if you have Celiac disease or irritable bowel syndrome (IBS). An unhealthy gastrointestinal tract may lead to further health complications. A recent study found that gut microbiota health practically relates to different systems and functions of the body.

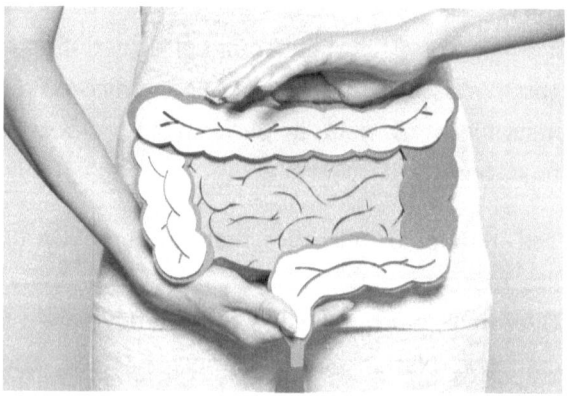

This interesting research found that the health of your GI tract may influence your risk of:

- Heart diseases
- Mental health issues, such as anxiety and depression
- Autoimmune diseases, including rheumatoid arthritis
- Metabolic diseases (chemical changes in your body causing obesity and diabetes)
- Osteoporosis and bone health (weak bones)

Your body is home to both harmful and helpful bacteria that live in the digestive tract. They not only support body functions, but promote overall good health. The harmful bacteria, may cause variety of diseases as their quantity is exceeded in the body. This is why you need a good balance and diversity for maintaining a healthy GI tract.

In order to do this, we not only need to look at our intake, we may need to supplement with a live culture of varied bacteria, known as Probiotics.

But what are Priobiotics?

A Brief History Of Probiotics

Long before one could recognize probiotic microorganisms, people consumed fermented food, such as yogurt, cheese, beer, and wine. Fermentation enhances the taste of food, but also makes it healthier. Romans treated intestinal problems with fermented milk without knowing how it works.

Even though our knowledge of specific microbes is only recent, fermentation and probiotics, and more importantly their benefits have been around for a long time. In 1800, the famous researcher Ilya Mechnikov observed Bulgarian people with relatively long-life spans despite harsh living climates and poverty. They consumed a diet rich in fermented milk and yogurt.

Later, in 1953, Werner Kollath, a German scientist, found some active substances in fermented foods. He further found these active substances are necessary for healthy development and growth. Stillwell and Lilly, after Werner, used the term 'Probiotic' to define organisms that help stimulate human growth in 1965.

Fuller, in 1993, explained probiotics as live microorganisms that benefit their host while improving intestinal bacterial balance. Modern science, with pioneering studies of Russian scientists and Nobel Laureates, Elie Metchnikoff, and Louis Pasteur, identified numerous functions of these microorganisms in the gut and how they affect human health. Louis Pasteur and Elie Metchnikoff conducted several studies at the Pasteur Institute to find how bacteria could reduce the effects of digestive disorders.

Research on probiotics accelerated over the next decades. Many controlled, randomized clinical studies identified the therapeutic and preventive role of probiotics on human health.

Chapter 2: Probiotics Are Real And Scientifically Proven

To understand the science behind underlying microbe treatments, you have to delve into the details of probiotics' reality. It is also important because bacteria and gut microbes have a long-term reputation for causing health complications.

There is a bulk of scientific evidence that suggests probiotics can not only treat medical conditions, but also prevent illnesses. A number of studies show that fermented food and probiotic supplements can help treat conditions like IBS, obesity, diarrhea, high cholesterol, and inflammatory disorders.

Let's navigate through the studies and literature to explore what probiotics are for and how do they help us!

Do Probiotics Really Help – Exploring The Other Side

Actually, probiotics may not work for everyone, many people find it hard to digest the idea of bacteria being a healthy or helpful organism. As mentioned earlier, bacteria are responsible for causing many diseases. People usually consider the benefits associated with probiotics as a tactic to create pure hype.

However, this is not the case. Many recent clinical studies show that quality probiotics with a diverse strain, can help balance the immune health as well as promoting healthy digestion. It is worth noting that your health, gene mechanism, age, and the microorganisms already present in your body, all affect the way probiotics work for your health.

If you think probiotics are not benefitting you, there might be several reasons, such as:

- You are not taking the right dose
- You are not following the directions given on the probiotic products
- The strain you are using is wrong for your symptoms
- You may have an immune disorder

That is to say, probiotics, if taken properly, it can help you in a number of ways and scientific evidence backs this up.

Let us look at these studies to explore the effectiveness of the health-friendly bacteria.

Researches And Scientific Evidence In Favor Of Probiotics

One of the studies published by the microbiology department of Sismanoglion General Hospital, Greece, in 2013, highlighted the functional significance of probiotics in the human body. The scientists of this study presented evidence supporting that gut-friendly bacteria in a daily diet will confer health benefits. The evidence showed the role of microbes in the treatment and prevention of certain medical conditions.

The study documented the effects of taking probiotics on several bowel disorders, including anti-biotic associated diarrhea, infectious diarrhea, and lactose intolerance. The study further highlighted the potential role of probiotics in treating other conditions. It laid a great deal of emphasis on incorporating probiotics in your dietary regime by increasing the consumption of dairy products and supplements.

A research article published in 2015 found the correlation between gut microbiota activity and common disorders, including inflammatory bowel diseases, hypertension, obesity, and hypercholesterolemia. The study aimed to find the role of probiotics in improving health and how they influence other healthy microbiota.

The Vivo clinical data of this study support the new health claims. Moreover, it built evidence that probiotics modulate the metabolism of the host while improving cholesterol metabolism, immune support, sensorimotor behavior, and skin health. The study mainly involved animals. The results showed that gut microbiota regulates inflammation, energy expenditure, glucose metabolism, and satiety.

The Maastricht V/Florence Consensus Report 2016 concluded that probiotics demonstrate promising results in reducing *H. pylori* (bacteria that can cause ulcers and sores on the stomach lining) side effects. Another meta-analysis based on randomized trials suggested that incorporating *H. Pylori* antibiotics with probiotic supplements to diet regime can help patients prevent these symptoms. This supplementation is helpful for people with severe eradication failure (treatment failure of *H. Pylori* removal).

A meta-analysis conducted in 2019 demonstrated that the gut microbiome plays an important role in treating radiation-induced diarrhea. It reinforces the intestinal function by strengthening the intestinal barrier, plus they improve innate immunity and stimulate intestinal repair mechanisms.

Several meta-analyses on specific probiotic strains concluded that they help patients reduce the duration and severity of infectious diarrhea, especially in children. Oral administration can shorten the duration of illness by one day. The claim underwent further testing through clinical trials on various probiotic strains, which showed consistent results. These trails also suggested that probiotics are effective and safe.

Mayo Clinic conducted two studies on the supporting functions of gut bacteria. The findings showed that microbes could be helpful in predicting the susceptibility of RA (Rheumatoid Arthritis). In addition, these gut-friendly bacteria can help medical professionals prevent and treat the disease.

Genome Medicine published a study in 2016 that analyzes the biomarker of RA. Researchers found out that the patients with RA had decreased diversity in the gut microbiome when compared with the control group.

Another study published by Arthritis & Rheumatology Medical Journal in 2016 found the benefits of the bacterium, *Prevotella cisticola*. The mice treated with this bacterium experienced less frequent and less severe symptoms of inflammation associated with Rheumatoid Arthritis.

In 2016, Plos One published a study that offered some evidence about a particular strain, *Lactobacillus johnsonii* that it may prevent some types of cancers. Researchers used this strain on mice associated with lymphomas, leukemia, and other forms of diseases. When the mice received treatment with *Lactobacillus johnsonii,* they developed lymphomas half quickly as compared with a control group.

The Journal of Applied Microbiology published a research in 2016 demonstrating the health benefits of *Akkermansia muciniphila*, a bacterial strain that can help patients prevent inflammation of heart muscles. If you ignore the symptoms of Myocarditis, they may lead to the build-up of fatty plaque in arteries. According to scientists, *Akkermansia muciniphila* could prevent this by blocking communication between cells in the gut lining. Due to this, fewer toxins and contaminants pass into the patient's bloodstream. This mechanism eventually results in reduced inflammation.

The University of Chicago published an online study in 2015 that found a particular strain of bacteria in mice digestive tracts that can help strengthen the immune system against melanoma tumor cells. Scientists compared the gains to anti-cancer medicines, called checkpoint inhibitors.

In summary, there are more and more studies on Gut health arising and many more than we've talked about here, as this information is relevant to today's population for many reasons. But we can see from this that Gut Health is an essential influencer in general health, and Probiotics play a vital role in it.

The Different Types Of Probiotics And Their Roles In The Human Body

The studies mentioned above provide a solid ground to show the benefits of probiotics for different diseases and their preventions. The live bacteria are superbly beneficial for several bodily functions, such as improving digestive health and stimulating brain activities. The live microorganisms not only treat or prevent illnesses but also promote overall wellness.

However, it is essential to understand that your bowel is the host to trillions of microbes. This is known as gut microbiome. The Harvard Medical School showed that every individual has a unique mix of bacteria. Some illnesses or medical conditions can influence the bacterial balance that may exacerbate digestive health. The good bacteria in the body produce specific proteins and enzymes to inhibit the harmful bacteria.

Knowing which bacteria are helpful for your health will help you achieve your health goals. Here is a list of scientifically proven probiotics and their role in the human body:

The two recognized genera in probiotics of a healthy gut microbiome are *Lactobacillus* and *Bifidobacterium*. These two genera of probiotics generally have an excellent track record when it comes to benefiting the human body.

Lactobacillus

It is one of the commonly consumed microorganisms that produce lactase. Lactase is an enzyme that the human body uses to break down milk sugar or lactose. Lactobacillus species are referred to as lactic acid bacteria. The bacteria help in decreasing the infectious bacteria and control their population. Lactobacillus bacteria are naturally found in:

- Mouth
- Small intestine

- Vagina

The strain of bacteria primarily colonizes in your small intestine. Whereas *Bifidobacterium*, colonizes in the colon and large intestine.

Lactobacillus Health Benefits To Human Body

As we mentioned earlier, not all strains of bacteria are considered beneficial for human health. Different strains have different functions that are beneficial for different bodily mechanisms. Let's go through some of the well-known strains and species of Lactobacillus and its benefits.

Lactobacillus Acidophilus

It is one of the most widely used strains of Lactobacillus bacterium. In the 1920s, this strain of bacteria was used in dairy products to promote digestive health.

In addition to supporting the digestive system of the human body, the strain helps people absorb nutrients and strengthen the immune system. Numerous studies have shown that acidophilus plays a crucial role in improving immune health and supporting vaginal health.

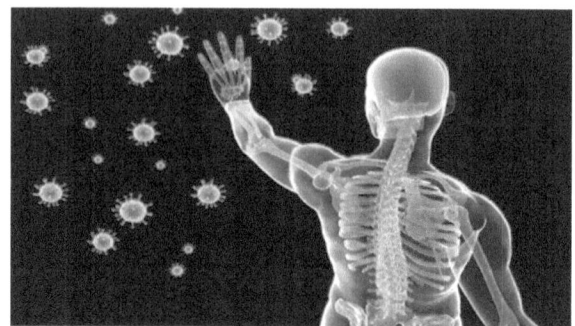

The most extended strain of *Lactobacillus acidophilus is DDS®-1*, which was discovered in 1950. This particular strain has an excellent quality to adhere to your intestinal wall, plus it is well-tolerated for almost all age groups and has impressive acid resistance. It typically offers the following benefits to the human body:

- Promotes immune system
- Helps in balancing the healthy gut microbiome
- Improves lactose digestion
- Helps in mild constipation

Lactobacillus Rhamnosus

This bacterial strain is naturally present in the human body. It is included in many dairy products. Many clinical studies have been conducted on *L. rhamnosus* and its benefits for children and adults, and this specific strain is linked to several health benefits, including:

- Healthy weight loss
- Healthy immune and digestive system
- Improved women health

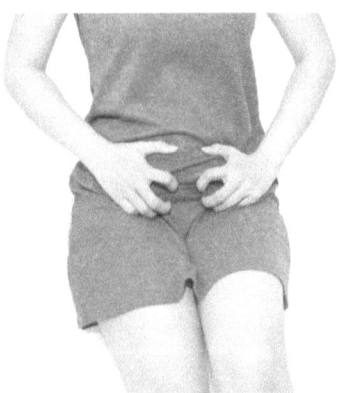

Lactobacillus Reuteri

This species is naturally existing probiotic found in the intestinal tract. It has a great bile and acid resistance, which allows it to stay, reproduce, and survive in the gut. The health benefit it provides to the human body includes:

- Improved oral health
- Healthy heart functions
- Improved women health

Lactobacillus Plantarum

Lactobacillus Plantarum is a unique strain of bacteria. It plays a vital role in producing antibodies that attack harmful bacteria in the GI tract. *L. Plantarum* can grow best at human body temperature and can easily survive the complicated digestive tract.

This useful bacterial has the following health benefits:

- Relieves digestion problems
- Fortifies immune system
- Alleviates occasional intestinal discomfort and bloating

Lactobacillus Gasseri

Lactobacillus gasseri BNR17 is a strain of bacteria that offers benefits related to weight management. It has been extensively studied and isolated from breast milk. Besides this, after several clinical trials and researches, the Korean FDA has declared these strains as functional ingredients for health and functional food.

Bifidobacterium Health Benefits To Human Body

Bifidobacteria - Probiotic Protection

Bifidobacteria are the most-studied probiotics. They comprise a large group of microorganisms with a plethora of overlapping benefits.

Bifidobacteria probiotics are mainly included in many dietary supplements. The probiotics are commonly used by the Japanese in their supplements to maintain the right quantity of healthy Bifidobacteria in the large intestine. Breastfeeding babies develop a high population of Bifidobacteria that support and promote their growth, plus the strain helps infants fend off many growth challenges by fortifying their immune system.

Another essential thing to keep in mind is that as you age, the number of Bifidobacteria decreases in the intestine. They are replaced by the harmful and less beneficial organisms that can multiply at high speed.

Using Bifidobacteria supplements for a healthy body has many benefits. Many studies have found that this particular strain of bacteria raises HDL cholesterol levels and lowers LDL in both animals and humans. This corresponding reduction of LDL cholesterol is a benefit in reducing the risk of cardiovascular diseases.

Bifidobacterium Lactis

This species of Bifidobacterium is extremely versatile and mostly found in dairy products like fermented milk and yogurt. This specific strain can:

- Support digestion
- Relieve constipation
- Support immune system

Bifidobacterium Bifidum

It is another common probiotic found in the human gastrointestinal tract. It naturally lives in the human gut since infancy. The strain is associated with plenty of benefits such as:

- Better lactose digestion
- Healthy food digestion
- Promoting a healthy immune system

Bifidobacterium Longum

This bacterial strain is a valuable protector of the intestinal walls, helping fight detrimental microorganisms. They help the body break down nutrients like lactose, proteins, and carbohydrates. Moreover, *B. longum* helps in:

- Relieving occasional constipation
- Promoting a healthy state of mind by relieving occasional stress
- Healthy digestion
- Strengthening the immune system

Bifidobacterium Infantis

As the name implies, this strain of bacteria is particularly advantageous and useful for infants' microbiome. It helps the human body:

- Minimize gastrointestinal distress caused by microbiome composition
- Aid in digesting breast milk
- Colonize the microbiome of babies with gut-friendly bacteria
- Utilize the sugar and nutrients in breast milk for healthy growth

As you can see that several strains of gut microbiota help in enhancing your overall health and well being. We will learn how these microbes formed an innate bond with us in upcoming chapters.

Chapter 3: The Development Of Probiotics In The Human Body

The last chapter provides adequate information about the clinical studies and researches on probiotics and how these tiny microorganisms can work with your body to promote and support your overall health.

The vital strains of gut bacteria contribute to improving digestive functions by replenishing your ecosystem of microbiome flora. They also strengthen immune health. That is to say; probiotics have a great ability to optimize bodily functions.

And when it comes to attaining healthy gut goals for children, the development of probiotics in the body is, without a doubt, one of the most critical steps. Know that, like many other vital organs in the body, the gut microbiome is essential for the human body to function correctly. The gut bacteria are nonexistent in the early phases of infancy. The first few years of childhood, however, experience extensive development of their size and roles.

How? Let's find out.

What Probiotics Mean For Infants And Growing Babies

Colonization of the digestive tract typically begins in the first few months after a child is born. This process continues in the first three years. After the age of three, the microbiota composition becomes the same as adult-like. Some of the recent studies have shown that some microorganisms colonize the baby's gut shortly after they are delivered when they interact with the environment.

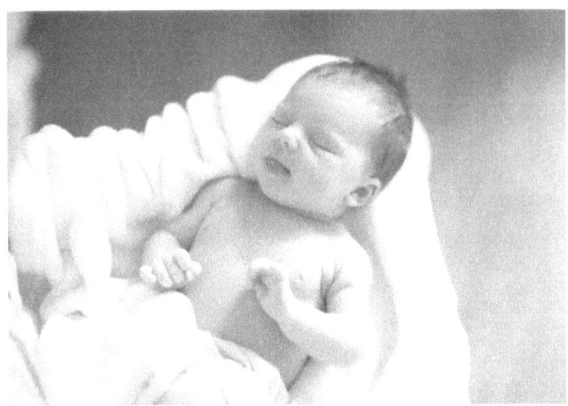

Another study showed that vaginally-delivered babies often have the same vaginal microbiota as their mothers have. However, babies delivered through Cesarean section do not have this tendency. It is because the method does not involve the natural process of transferring bacteria through the birth canal. As a result, babies delivered through the cesarean way have a naturally lower diversity of gut bacteria.

This is one of the reasons why many child health experts consider vaginal deliveries helpful in colonizing the healthy bacteria in the baby's gut. A bulk of evidence and clinical trials has demonstrated the benefits of probiotics for the healthy development of the children. Probiotics are considered safe for babies because they support healthy development. Daily incorporation of probiotic supplementation to baby's diet can help:

- Support a healthy and active immune system; especially in the babies delivered through C-section
- Reduce the need to use antibiotic medicines and treatments in babies attending daycare

- Promote healthy gastrointestinal functions
- Reduce symptoms of colic
- Reduce the risk associated with allergies and severe skin infections
- Reduce gastrointestinal distress

According to the latest study published in NCIB, babies who are given probiotic supplements could improve fecal biochemistry. Researchers measured several samples of poops, which show a 79 percent increase in Bifidobacteria. It is incredibly beneficial for improving digestive health in babies. Furthermore, the researchers further found a significant decrease in harmful bacteria in babies' digestive, intestinal tract.

Bifidobacteria are also considered beneficial for lowering the pH levels in the intestine. The low pH level makes a suitable environment for probiotics to thrive and eliminate harmful bacteria. Besides that, when the pH level is low, it helps kill pathogenic bacteria in the gastrointestinal tract. Still, years of research are required to pin down whether or not altering the baby's gut with diverse microbes can help reduce the number of diseases. However, some current studies found probiotics useful for some medical conditions in children. For example, a recent study shows that probiotics can help treat and prevent diarrhea in babies taking antibiotics. Another research has shown that supplementing babies with probiotics may reduce their crying. Many pediatric gastroenterologists recommend probiotics for treating digestive issues like diarrhea.

Thus, there is no question that probiotics are not only safe for growing babies but can boost their immunity. However, remember that probiotics have many different strains that may have clinical effects. Considering the safety profiles of different strains of probiotics is a necessary step as well as consulting a healthcare professional before you give it your baby.

Probiotics And Its Effects On Various Body Systems

The current studies and researches on probiotics have proven that their benefits are not confined to gut health only. And that includes everything from your cognition to the respiratory system. The gut microbiome and disease are interrelated. Let's go through the effects of probiotics on your various body systems.

Probiotics And The Nervous System – The Gut-Brain Axis

No matter how bizarre it may sound to you, your gut bacteria may enhance your cognition. According to research, there is a connection between your GI tract and the brain. This partnership between gut and brain is labeled as the "gut-brain axis". The link is established via biochemical signaling between your digestive tract and nervous system. This part of the system, known as the enteric nervous system, forms a connection between gut and brain with the help of the Vagus nerve-the longest nerve in your body.

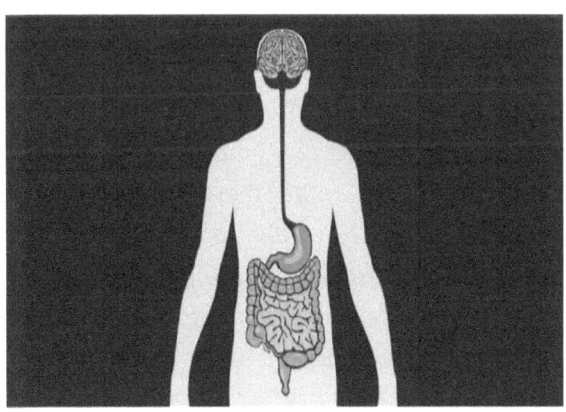

That is why the gut is often called as your second brain. It produces plenty of the neurotransmitters as your brain does. These neurotransmitters include gamma-aminobutyric acid, serotonin, and dopamine, all play a pivotal role in managing stress and regulating mood. According to estimation, the human digestive tract makes 90 percent of the serotonin in the body.

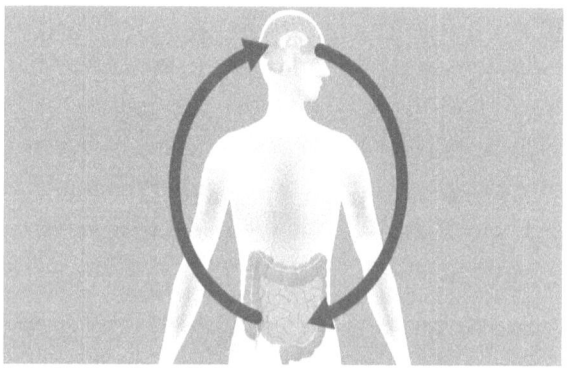

If you have ever experienced an inflammatory flare in your GI tract or stomach during stressful situations, it is due to these transmitters. It happens when the brain senses trouble and sends a flight response to the gut. That is why many people experience digestive problems when dealing with depression or anxiety.

Probiotics And Cognitive Functions

Several studies have shown how the gut-brain axis can regulate the brain and digestion activities in the body. The same studies have demonstrated the impact of gut-friendly bacteria on cognition. A study conducted in the UK on probiotics found a significant improvement in long and short-term memories of rats when they were given a solution of Bifidobacterium and Lactobacillus. Some of the robust improvements were also noticed in their spatial navigation.

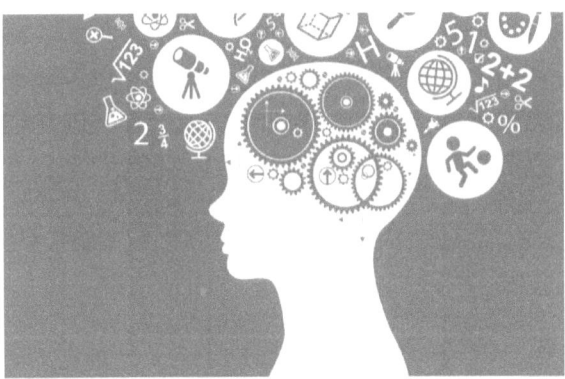

Apart from this clinical analysis, many animal trials are showing how probiotics can help reverse severe cognitive impairment. For example, obesity is linked with a decline in cognition. Chinese researchers found many probiotic supplements useful in restoring normal cognitive functions in people struggling with obesity.

In addition to this, according to Dr. Chyn Boon Wong - Research Associate at Morinaga Nutritional Foods, Singapore, found that probiotics play a significant role in preventing severe cognitive impairments such as Alzheimer's Disease (AD). It is one of the irreversible neurodegenerative diseases that result in slow cognitive impairment and may lead to dementia if not treated on time. Even though AD has become one of the most prevalent cognitive impairments in aging people, there is no clinically therapeutic strategy for treatment and prevention.

Dr. Chyn conducted a study that shows live microorganisms confer many benefits for patients when they ingest them in a sufficient amount. Some probiotics strains influence the central nervous system as well as behavior through the microbiota-gut-brain axis. Increasing evidence from various clinical studies demonstrated that microbes contain a therapeutic potential that can prevent AD and other cognitive impairments.

Probiotics And The Metabolism

The way your gut microbes metabolize primary acidic solutions to secondary acidic solution significantly affect the metabolism. During this process, the *farnesoid X* receptors are activated that help control fat in the body and balance blood sugar levels. That means your gut bacteria may have to do more with your obesity than you might have thought.

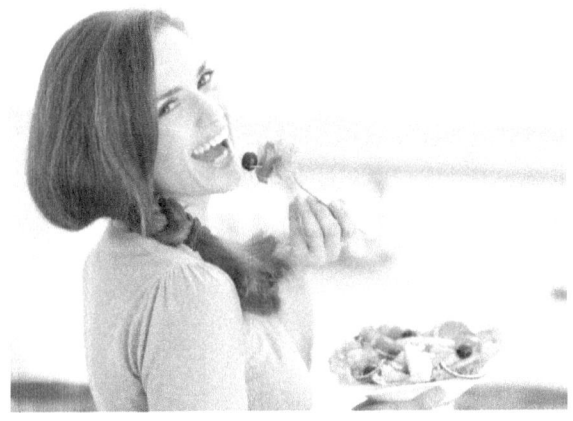

Not only this, probiotics can help you treat many non-alcoholic liver diseases and type 2 diabetes. When you administer a sufficient amount of probiotics, it enables you to improve metabolic health by reducing waist circumference and body fat mass. Inflammation in the stomach and liver is another metabolic disease that can be prevented with adequate intake of probiotics.

Metabolism has a vital role in maintaining your weight. Many studies have shown that probiotics can help people prevent obesity. A currently conducted meta-analysis on the effects of probiotics supplementation on overweight people found an optimal improvement of glucose metabolism and plasma lipids in their bodies. The probiotics supplements can increase the short-chain fatty acids (produced by bacteria) and decrease Lipopolysaccharide (LPS). As a result, LPS induced inflammation decreases, and tissues are relieved of trouble.

Besides this, probiotics can help reduce several opportunistic pathogens and metabolites by decreasing fat accumulation in the body. An adequate dose of probiotics improves insulin sensitivity and increases gastrointestinal peptide. This overall mechanism promotes metabolic homeostasis to keep the body in a healthy condition.

Probiotics And The Immune System

One of the most exciting locations for a bacterial fiesta is your gut. The food with its nutrients does not directly enter your bloodstream. It makes its way through the digestive tract and gut wall. This is what makes your GI tract a vital player for the immune system of your body.

The friendly bacteria in your gut fortify the body's immunity and keep dangerous toxins and potentially dangerous substances outside, plus the probiotics help body organs absorb the goodness from the food and drinks you consume. Moreover, the gut microbiome guards the intestinal wall and lets the beneficial bacteria pass. Your microbiota not only strengthens the gut wall, but it also competes with harmful bacteria and regulates the immune-inflammatory responses. The latest study found that probiotics can even withstand the harsh conditions of the GI tract. They can survive high alkaline and acidic levels of bile salt and gastric juices and can promote immune health by inhibiting pathogenic bacteria.

Moreover, one of the potential advantages of probiotics is that they trigger immune cells to help the body fight against tumors. Of course more study needs to be done, but the potential benefits on cancerous cells is an exciting area of exploration.

Furthermore, it serves as an immunity booster for an unborn infant when a pregnant mother takes probiotics during pregnancy. It helps infants avoid detrimental immune-mediated disorders that include type-1 diabetes, eczema, and asthma.

Probiotics can boost the integrity of mucous membranes of the colon. Also, probiotics stimulate antibodies to reduce the duration and incidents of digestion problems, like diarrhea, by strengthening the immune functions.

Probiotics And The Respiratory System

As we have seen, probiotic bacteria can be beneficial in preventing a wide variety of human diseases and medical conditions; in particular but perhaps less obvious, many respiratory diseases.

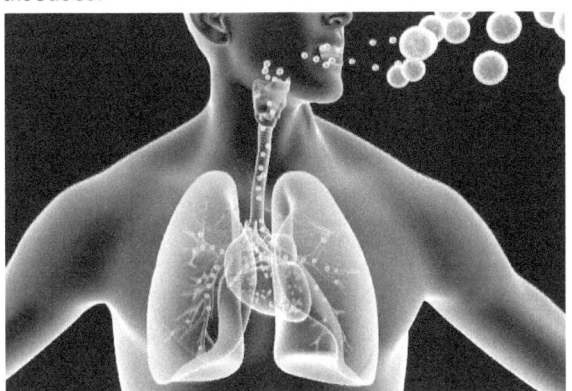

Scientists have used several microbe-based therapeutic approaches to treat respiratory infections and asthma. A recent study, for example, suggested that probiotics bacteria can minimize the duration and risk of respiratory infections.

Furthermore, a meta-analysis from western, Lawson Health Research Institute, Laval University, and Utrecht University found that using probiotics may eliminate almost 2.3 million days of respiratory tract infections per year. This is a staggering statistic and would have a significant impact on the lives of many people.

Acute viral respiratory infection is one of the most common heath issues. On average, babies and infants experience 4 to 8 respiratory infections yearly. The significant pathogens and viruses that cause these infections include rhinoviruses, respiratory syncytial virus, enterovirus, adenovirus, and parainfluenza virus. Not only this, more than 250 viruses similar to these can cause acute respiratory infections.

Probiotics, such as *Lactobacillus rhamnosus*, when combined with other probiotics, play an essential role in reducing the risk of URI (Upper Respiratory Infections) risks, especially in children. A recently conducted systematic review highlighted some favorable outcomes of probiotic use in reducing the growth of Rhinovirus and coronavirus significantly.

The pathology and physiology of the gastrointestinal tract and respiratory tract are related to each other. This similarity justifies the reasons why the dysfunction of one organ can affect the other one.

For instance, smoking is one of the major risk factors of Inflammatory Bowel Disease (IBD) and Chronic Obstructive Pulmonary Disease

(COPD). It can increase the risks associated with Crohn's disease. Probiotics, such as *Lactobacillus, Saccharomyces, and Bifidobacterium* regulate the inflammatory immune response in both the GI tract and respiratory system.

Some Diseases That Probiotics May Help Cure

The trillions of microorganisms found in your intestinal tract are of the hottest subjects in medicine. With the health benefits probiotics claim to provide, it is no surprise why they have become must-have food supplements to boost overall health. These tiny microbes can be of great help in maintaining a balance of healthy and harmful bacteria in your gut.

This is one of the reasons why probiotics gained popularity and more attention in the medical domain. Many practicing physicians and pediatrics show tremendous interest in studying how intestinal microbes can help patients treat health problems.

So far, the studies show mixed results as some researchers found probiotics beneficial for health, while others were finding it not so valuable. However, there are some medical conditions that currently have strong and positive scientific evidence to use and support the use of probiotics. Some of them include:

- **Crohn's Disease**

Crohn's is an inflammatory disease that affects the gastrointestinal tract. People with this disease experience many uncomfortable to debilitating digestive problems. Luckily, probiotics can help patients overcome the symptoms of Crohn's disease, whether patients take probiotics in the form of supplements or eat food that has probiotics such as kefir, yogurt, and miso. (Not all probiotic supplements are same, not all yogurts are same. Ex: Greek yogurt cultured in jar has higher probiotics than mainstream flavored yogurts.) It may reduce inflammation in the stomach significantly.

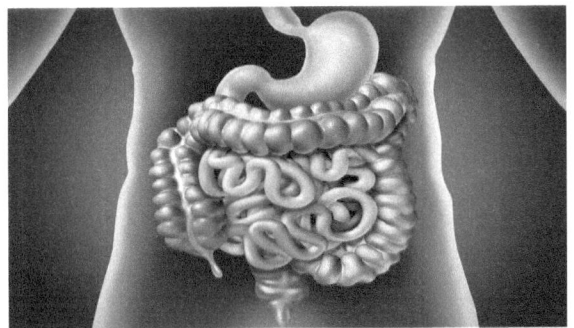

According to studies, patients who have Crohn's disease have an altered microbiome. It means that even their regular microbiome makeup in their gastrointestinal tract is unbalanced. The use of probiotics may help these patients reduce their symptoms by broadening the variety microbiome, which in turn would result in significantly reducing irregular immune response.

The helpful bacteria minimize severe symptoms associated with Crohn's disease, including upset stomach, gastrointestinal irritation, and diarrhea. Incorporating probiotic foods into the diet is also an excellent idea to promote gut health and reduce symptoms of Crohn's disease.

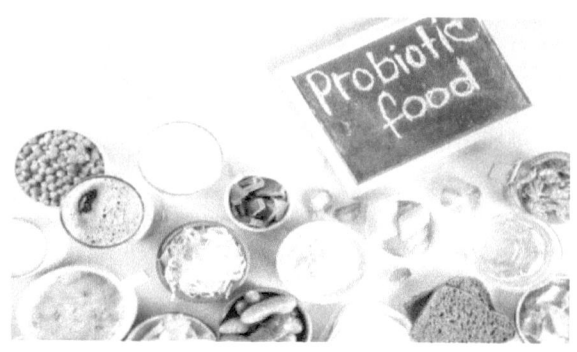

Another research conducted in 2014 showed that gut microbes could effectively improve the function of the intestinal barrier and cytokines quantity. The cytokines are anti-inflammatory chemical compounds in the GI tract. The study concluded that probiotics have excellent promising therapeutic properties to minimize the symptoms of inflammatory bowel disease and Crohn's disease.

- **Irritable Bowel Syndrome (IBS)**

Tied to the same group of digestive health problems discussed in the previous section, IBS is one of the chronic disorders that cause abdominal pain and change in bowel movements. It also causes gas, bloating, and diarrhea. IBS is common nowadays due to a reduction in healthy dietary intake and an increase   in   "fast   foods."

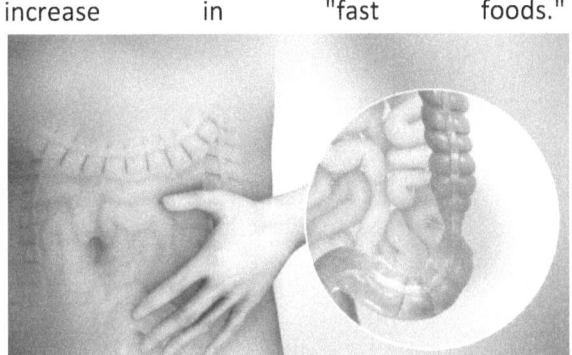

There is growing evidence on the positive effects of probiotics to reduce discomfort and symptoms caused by IBS. The digestive disorder is linked to causing changes in patients' gut flora.

For instance, if you experience the symptoms of IBS, you might have a lower number of strains of Bifidobacterium and Lactobacillus in your gastrointestinal tract. Not only this, the disorder may increase the amount of *Streptococcus* and *Clostridium*, which are harmful bacteria in the gut. Research on IBS showed that 84 percent of people with IBS suffer from harmful bacterial overgrowth in the small intestine. Probiotics are linked to the following improved symptoms of IBS as they can:

- Inhibit disease-causing bacterial growth

- Enhance the barrier function of the gut
- Slow down bowel movement
- Reduces inflammation
- Reduce gas production thereby decreasing the severity of bloating
- Reduce the GI tract's sensitivity to gas buildup

However, it is essential to keep in mind that not all microbes function in the same way. Different probiotics have different strains, and they may vary in health effects. Certain Probiotics, such as yeast, can help IBS patients restore gut flora balance in plenty of ways. Adding food made of yeast to the diet can reduce inflammation caused by IBS and speeds up the metabolism.

A comprehensive review conducted in 2016 concluded that using probiotics may help in treating IBS symptoms. The study found that specific probiotic strains have the potential to lower the symptoms of IBS. Lactobacillus, Bifidobacterium, and *Saccharomyces* have shown promising results. These strains helped 214 test patients of IBS reduce bloating and pain. A German study treated 297 IBS patients with a two-strain probiotic liquid called *Pro-Symbioflor*. The supplement reduced 50 percent of general symptoms associated with IBS in patients, including inflammation and abdominal pain.

However, more clinical data and evidence are required to prove the consistent mechanism these probiotic strains use to ward off the symptoms but the symptoms are promising.

- **Obesity**

Obesity is a growing epidemic worldwide and is linked to the rise of many other diseases. As a common problem globally, there is much study of the healthy gut microbiome and its connection to obesity. The evidence so far has demonstrated that the microbes present in the gastrointestinal tract affect energy regulation and nutrient acquisition, which play a crucial role in weight gain and development of obesity.

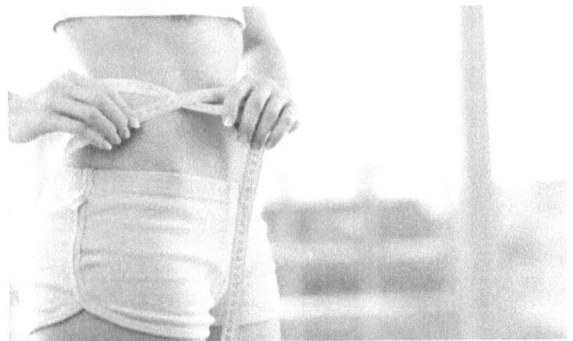

As already mentioned that beneficial bacteria present in your gut help break down food for easy digestion. These bacteria will extract the essential nutrients from the foods you consume. However, if your digestive system is not healthy, it can lead to a condition called dysbiosis, which indicates an imbalance in the GI microbes.

A study conducted in 2015 suggested that people who suffer from weight gain problems or obesity have imbalanced gut microbiota. This imbalanced gut flora can be one of the causes of obesity. The researchers of this study further found some factors that cause changes in human gut flora and lead it to obese patterns. The factors include:

- High-calorie or high-fat diet
- Use of sweeteners
- Disturbed diurnal rhythm

Luckily, the strain of *Lactobacillus amylovorus and Lactobacillus fermentum* may help with healthy weight management. The bacterial strain is present in yogurt when combined with a healthy diet that helps obese people reduce 3 to 4 percent body fat.

In a study, researchers examined Lactobacillus gasseri's effects on fat loss. The study participants who consumed fermented milk products along with a regular healthy diet were able to lose 8.5 percent belly fat over 12 to 13 weeks. The results suggest that probiotics can be immensely helpful for weight loss among people suffering from obesity.

- **Diarrhea**

Many clinical studies show that adding probiotics to the diet of both children and adults may help treat and prevent diarrhea. They are specifically beneficial when their antibiotic course starts. Antibiotic-associated diarrhea is one of the common side effects of taking high medicine doses. The medicines are powerful enough to wipe out both healthy and harmful bacteria in the intestinal tract, and that may disturb the healthy microbial balance of intestine. This condition causes diarrhea in more than 30 percent of people who receive treatment.

As we now know, Probiotics replenish the lost friendly microbes, and that may help patients suffering from antibiotic-associated diarrhea. Also, they restore gastrointestinal balance.

According to medical professionals, intestines need time to recover from the effects of antibiotics. Most of them recommend that patients should continue the use of probiotics in their diets for at least one month after they finish their antibiotic course.

The Rotavirus is one of the common causes of troubled tummy or upset stomach in children. Some Recent studies on diarrhea in babies show promising results of using probiotics.

The bacteria strains of *Lactobacillus rhamnosus and lactobacillus reuteri* and probiotic yeast are very useful when it comes to cutting bouts of infection by half a day. Doctors often use a mix of different probiotics to treat diarrhea in children.

Moreover, people who suffer from severe colon inflammation and life-threatening diarrhea can also benefit from probiotic doses. *C. difficile* can cause both these conditions. Consuming probiotics may help people fighting this infection. Some clinical trials also suggest that usage of probiotics can stop diarrhea from coming back by strengthening the lining of the stomach and the small intestine.

- **Ulcerative Colitis**

Ulcerative Colitis is another persistent digestive disorder that causes ulceration in the colon. These ulcers are sores, and inflammation is caused by a genetic mutation, which in turn allows the harmful bacteria present to irritate the intestines, which results in a disruption of the protective epithelial lining of the stomach and small intestine.

Currently, there are treatments but no cure for this condition. Surgery and medication may help, but flare-ups are regularly experienced afterward. Promising results have been found with the use of Probiotics to help relieve the symptoms of UC.

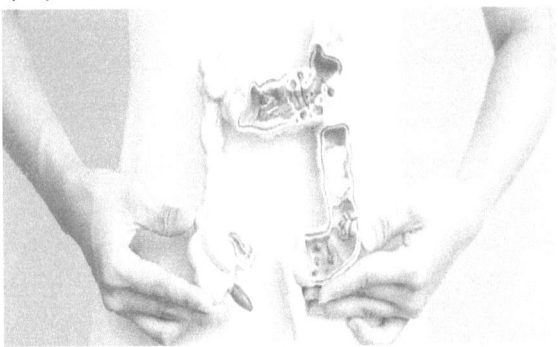

Patients can experience Flare-ups and inflammation even after surgery or medication.

So how do gut microbes can help relieve UC symptoms?

Probiotics have optimal effects on Ulcerative Colitis. The evidence on UC's treatment showed that friendly bacteria could help create a balance in gut flora. They reduce the number of harmful bacteria, thereby reducing the incidents of inflammation and abdominal discomfort. Doctors recommend patients experiencing UC symptoms to include healthy bacteria or probiotics in the diet to keep the gastrointestinal tract healthy.

Adding fermented products high in natural microflora to diet is very useful for relieving inflammation and other symptoms associated with Ulcerative Colitis.

- **Vaginal Infections**

Consuming probiotics is an excellent solution to improve vaginal health. The health experts identified plenty of potential benefits of gut microbes for vaginal health. The probiotic strain *L. acidophilus* can help women prevent vaginal imbalance. The vaginal fluids are moderately acidic, with a pH between 3.8 and 4.5. If the pH balance is disturbed, several opportunistic pathogens can cause an infection resulting in

Bacterial Vaginosis (BV). Several species of lactobacilli are usually present inside the vagina, which maintain the optimum pH levels and reduce the risk of infections.

But, if lactobacilli, with some other microbes, overgrow, it may lead to an imbalance in vaginal bacteria. There can be a number of reasons for lactobacilli overgrowth. Precisely, women suffer from this vaginal infection if they:

- Experience hormonal changes
- Irregularity in period
- Do not maintain hygiene habits
- Have unprotected sex

And that imbalance of microbes in the vagina may result in:

- Discomfort
- Discharge
- Unusual odor
- Itching
- Yeast infections
- Favorable environment for Trichomoniasis

To prevent all these vaginal problems, maintaining balance in the bacterial strain is imperative. By consuming whole foods and probiotic supplements, women can keep these vaginal issues at bay. The bacteria stick to vaginal surfaces and serve as a barrier, not allowing harmful bacteria to pass through. Besides this, *Lactobacillus* adheres to dangerous bacteria and kills them.

• **Bladder Cancer Recurrence**

Probiotics are so far touted for a plethora of benefits when it comes to treating medical conditions, including weight loss, autoimmune disorders, vaginal imbalance, and digestive disorders.

Surprisingly, a large area of clinical research covers probiotics and its effects on non-muscle bladder cancer (after treatment). Researchers have conducted several clinical trials on the bacterial strain *Lactobacillus casei Shirota* that is only present in "Yakult" (a Japanese fermented milk beverage).

The growing evidence on this specific probiotic suggests that it can prevent the reoccurrence of bladder cancer if consumed in a large amount. Probiotics influence the action of Dendritic cells of the immune system in the prevention of cancer. The dendritic cells are the primary recruiters and mobilizers of Natural Killer (NK) cells. These NK cells play a significant role in reducing the risk of cancer recurrence.

If consumed correctly and in enough quantities, probiotics may prevent the risk of this cancer along with the recurrence.

Chapter 4: Prebiotics Are Not Probiotics

So far, we learnet that the way we live and what we eat makes a significant difference in our gut health and immune system.

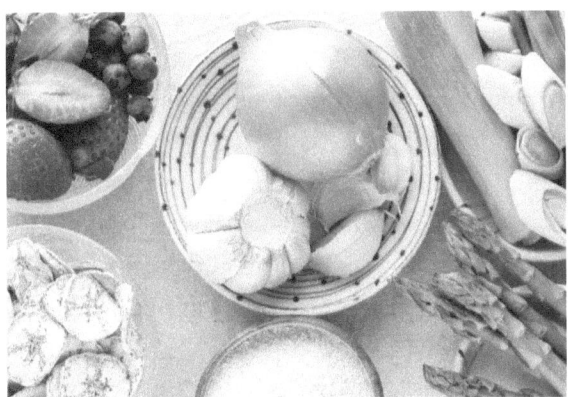

To improve gut health, it is substantially important to understand the difference between probiotics and prebiotics. Learning about probiotics alone is not enough to strengthen overall immunity, along with your gut health.

Prebiotics also have a vital role to play when it is about conferring health benefits. In this chapter, we will shed some light on the vital role that the relatively new "Prebiotics" play in our gut health, and how they affect the gut microbiome.

What Are Prebiotics?

Although both probiotics and prebiotics are essential for your health, it is important to understand that both have different roles to play.

Probiotics are the live microbes found in fermented food and supplements, providing plenty of health benefits. On the other hand, Prebiotics are the different substances found in carbs and fibers that are usually indigestible for humans. However, the friendly bacteria in the gastrointestinal tract feed on this fiber.

International Scientific Association for Probiotics & Prebiotics (ISAPP) states that prebiotics are typically a substrate that your host microorganisms use to confer health benefits.

While probiotics are the microorganisms, the term prebiotics refers to food compounds that help these microorganisms grow. Many studies have established that if you increase the consumption of food that's rich in prebiotics, you can:

- Regulate your blood sugar level
- Improve colon health
- Boost calcium absorption

Benefits Of Prebiotics For Human Health

Since the given definitions clarify the confusion you might have regarding the roles of prebiotics and probiotics, let us see how they are beneficial for your health.

- **Boost Bacterial Composition Of Hind Gut**

As prebiotics have tons of health-promoting properties, they are the markers of a healthy microbiota. Prebiotics have a target of improving dietary stimulation. For example, prebiotics help in increasing the number of *Lactobacilli*, which may help reduce severe mucosal inflammation in the gastrointestinal tract.

Not only this, it plays an essential role in digesting lactose, especially in lactose-intolerant individuals.

- **Help Reduce Cancer Risk**

Adequate consumption of prebiotics may help reduce the number of cancer cells and free radicals in the body. Particularly, colon cancer increases toxins in the body that are difficult to remove quickly. Some recently conducted studies indicated a decrease in cancer and tumor cells in the people who had a prebiotics-rich diet.

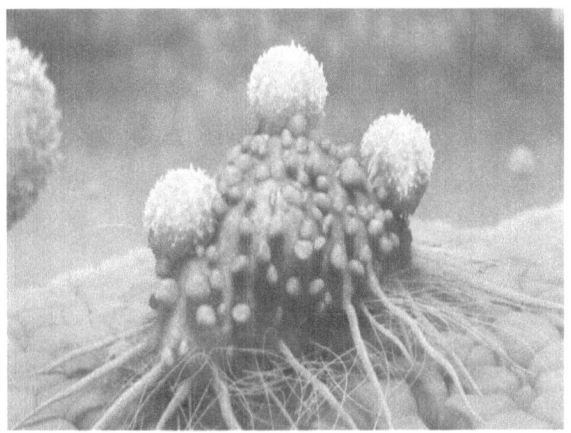

- **Help You Control Blood Pressure**

The one prominent health benefit you get from incorporating foods rich in prebiotics into your diet is controlled blood pressure. Prebiotics help your body balance electrolyte and mineral levels. As a result, your blood pressure remains stable.

- **Improve Nutrient Absorption**

Remember that the composition of a healthy microbiome depends on prebiotics. Without prebiotics, probiotics will not exist.

Prebiotics help microorganisms in your body recolonize in your gut. It is worth noting that when the human body absorbs nutrients properly, it shuts down its autoimmune responses. The condition helps the body convert food into energy.

Moreover, prebiotics also strengthens the bones by absorbing nutrients, such as calcium and magnesium.

- **Help To Maintain Hormone Health**

Plenty of recent studies have linked gut health to mood regulation. When you include prebiotics-rich food or supplement into your diet, they improve the chemical composition of hormones. This eventually helps alleviate mood disorders, such as depression and anxiety.

- **Improve Immune Functions And Reduces Inflammation**

Both probiotics and prebiotics help improve bowel movements, which reduce infections and allergies while strengthening immunity. As mentioned before, prebiotics helps the human body with nutrient absorption. This helps the immune system in improving its functions. It also relieves inflammation caused by digestive disorder by increasing the levels of healthy bacteria.

- **Decrease Risk Of Heart Diseases**

Prebiotics can help decrease the risk of cardiovascular diseases. If you consume your recommended dose of prebiotics (about 5-6 grams), it reduces glycation, which is one of the critical causes of increased free radicals in your body. Free radicals lead to oxidative stress in the healthy cells, such as proteins, DNA, and immune cells – and of course, the gut microbiome. Prebiotics have a hypo-cholesterolemic effect on the human body that combats the symptoms associated with cardiovascular diseases.

Best Sources Of Prebiotics

We now can see the importance of prebiotics for gut microbes. The indigestible fiber feeds the good bacteria in your gut to keep them thriving. Working together with probiotics, they create balance in the gastrointestinal tract while promoting overall health.

Fortunately, you can enjoy the potential health benefits of prebiotics by adding delicious foods, which are rich in prebiotics, to your diet to feed your gut bacteria.

Here is a list of some organic prebiotics-rich foods to help you improve your wellbeing:

- **Asparagus**

The nutrient-rich vegetable is one of the fantastic prebiotic. Not only does it promote healthy gut bacteria, but it also helps reduce inflammation. This vegetable is rich in healthy vitamins, minerals, and antioxidants. Many studies have shown its benefits in preventing some forms of cancer, particularly liver cancer.

Enjoy steamed asparagus or make it a part of your green salad - this delicious and healthy vegetable is an excellent add-on to your pantry.

- **Bananas**

The creamy fruit is high in vitamins, minerals, and fibers. It is readily available at any time of the year. According to experts, unripe bananas make a good source of prebiotics. They are useful for not only increasing beneficial gut bacteria but also improving muscle regeneration and reducing bloating.

Adding banana to your daily diet is an ideal way to satiate your untimely sugar cravings. You can make fruit salads with bananas and a variety of smoothies.

- **Onions**

This nutrient-dense and versatile vegetable comes with a sufficient amount of prebiotics, flavonoids, and antioxidants. Onions can boost your healthy gut flora, strengthen the immune system, and improve cardiovascular health.

- **Garlic**

The herb is popular for its medicinal uses and offers many antimicrobial benefits. Garlic has a rich quantity of prebiotics to aid digestion and keep gastrointestinal diseases at bay.

It is best to eat garlic in raw form. Make sure you leave it for ten minutes after crushing or chopping for activating the enzymes that provide fantastic health benefits.

Best Fermented Foods For Healthy Gut Microbiome

Although probiotics from supplements are the perfect way to obtain them, you can also get them from a variety of fermented foods.

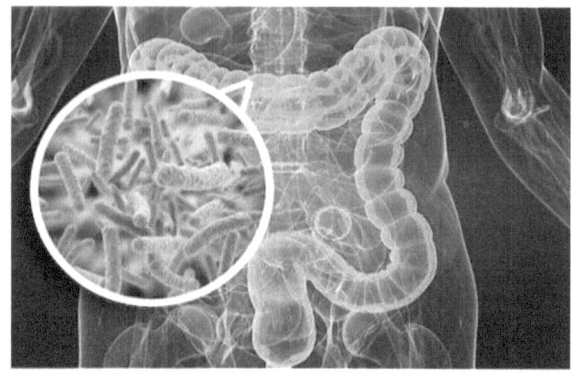

You can try some of the given options:

Yogurt

You might know that yogurt is the best source of getting probiotics to maintain your gut health. Probiotics come mainly from milk, fermented by beneficial bacteria, such as *Bifidobacteria* and Lactic acid bacteria.

Yogurt has tons of other health benefits that include improved bone health and heart health. It also helps people relieve many symptoms of diarrhea and IBS. Yogurt makes one of the best probiotic-rich foods for people suffering from lactose intolerance.

Kefir

Kefir grains are used to prepare delicious fermented-probiotic milk. It is important to note that Kefir grains are different from cereal grains. They are like cultures of yeast and lactic acid and their shape is like florets of cauliflower. Interestingly, kefir contains plenty of major strains of healthy bacteria that make it a potent source of diverse probiotics.

Tempeh

Tempeh is another great fermented product that helps you get your maximum proportion of probiotics. It is a soy product made by fermentation of soybeans. A controlled fermentation process makes the soybeans into a cake form. A specific fungal species, Rhizopus oligsporus is used in fermenting the soybeans.

Look for Appendix for probiotic Supplements

Chapter 5: The Best Recipes Packed With Gut-healthy Probiotics

We've discussed in depth the positive health benefits of incorporating probiotics and prebiotics to your diet to keep a super healthy gut microbiome. From helping constipation, stomach distress and various other healthy complications, the benefits are clear.

This chapter we now look at some easy and scrumptious recipes to create yourself to maximize your probiotic intake, and incorporate them into your diet regime.

Kombucha Tea

Kombucha tea has tons of promising benefits with an underlying sweetness that remains on your taste buds for the whole day. The tea requires fermentation with "SCOBY," which stands for "Symbiotic Culture." It is a jelly-like substance that floppy and slippery. It is used for the fermentation process.

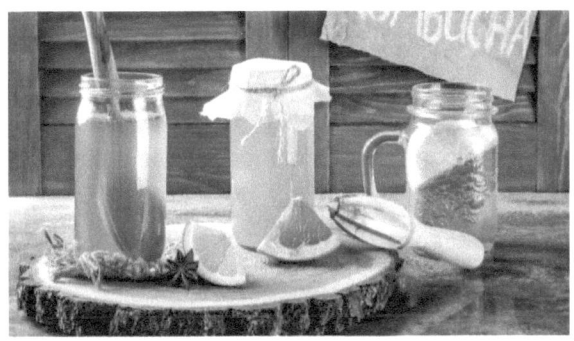

Ingredients

For one gallon batch of Kombucha tea

- 8 to 9 tea bags (non-herbal or unflavored) or you can also use loose tea (two tea bags)
- 1-3 cups starter liquid (available on Amazon or in your nearest local food store)
- 1 SCOBY
- Tea towel (breathable fabric)
- 1-gallon glass jar
- 1 cup of sugar

Directions

- Boil four cups of water and add tea. Steep the mixture for 10 minutes
- Remove all the tea bags - add sugar and stir until it is dissolved

- Transfer this tea liquid to gallon container and fill with water
- Place SCOBY and pour the starter liquid
- Cover this container with a breathable cloth
- Keep the jar at 78 to 85 degrees Fahrenheit for perfect breeding of bacteria
- Once prepared, you can use this Kombucha liquid for the next batch

Try adding your favorite flavors, or a delicious combination of them to create your own tailored recipes.

Try Lemon, Ginger, Tart-Cherry, Raspberry, Blackberry & Thyme, Fresh Fruit Puree

Coconut Milk Yogurt

Yogurt coconut milk is an amazing dairy-free alternative that you can make at home easily. The flavor of this naturally prepared non-dairy product is delicious. You can control the sweetness and sourness of yogurt by allowing minimum or maximum fermentation time for coconut milk.

Ingredients
How to make coconut milk:

- 2 ½ cups of unsweetened coconut
- 5 cups of heated and then cooled water

How To Make Coconut Milk Yogurt:
- 3 cups of coconut milk
- ½ cup coconut yogurt or 4 to 5 probiotic capsules
- 1 tbsp bovine gelatin

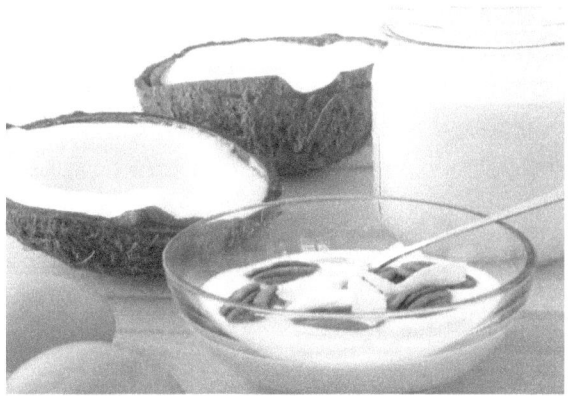

Directions
- Blend water and coconut with Vitamix blender until it is finely blended
- Strain the liquid using a fine sieve - squeeze out the remaining liquid with the help of a nut milk bag
- Add ½ cup of coconut yogurt or probiotic capsules (break them) to milk and stir it until it gets smooth

- Place this mixture in the bowl of hot water and leave it overnight
- Your coconut milk will begin to separate when you remove it from the bowl - add gelatin and stir to make it smoother
- Refrigerate for at least 2 hours before use

Almond Milk Kefir

Homemade almond milk kefir is creamier and richer in taste. Also, it contains many beneficial organisms and enzymes because it does not go through pasteurization. If you do not have kefir grains to make almond milk, you can use a kefir starter culture. The starter culture will be available in your local food store or you can get that through online.

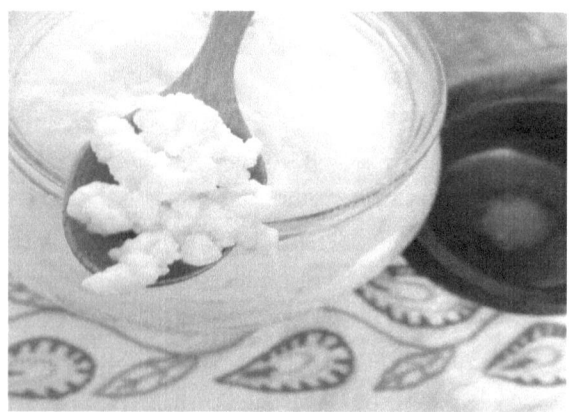

Ingredients

- 2 ½ cups almond milk
- 4 tbsp coconut sugar
- 1 direct-set starter culture package

Directions

- Mix milk with sugar and direct-set culture in a jar
- Cover with a lid (permeable)
- Allow the mixture to culture for 24-48 hours at room temperature
- During the process, the almond milk will separate into a creamier liquid layer
- Swirl or stir the two together
- When the milk gets tangy, it is cultured
- Store in the fridge or consume immediately

Kimchi

Kimchi is a Korean recipe made of fermented veggies such as radish and napa cabbage. It goes with just about everything, including noodles and meat. Whether it is fermented or fresh, it tastes great and contains loads of probiotics.

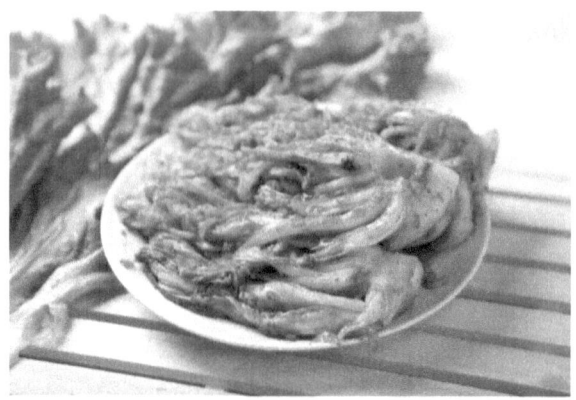

Ingredients

- 1 tbsp coarse sea salt
- Water
- 2 Napa cabbage, cut into 2-inch wedges,
- One garlic (peeled and separated)
- 1 piece of ginger root
- 1/4 cup Korean salted shrimps
- 1 radish (grated)
- Green onions or scallions (one bunch)
- 1/4 cup chili powder
- 1 tsp sugar
- Sesame oil
- Sesame seeds

Directions

- Soak cabbage pieces in salted water for four hours
- Combine shrimp, ginger, garlic, and shrimp and blend them finely
- Combine green onions, radish, salt, chili powder, mustard greens, and garlic and toss gently
- Drain water from the cabbage and stuff it with radish mixture
- Start with large leaves to small leaves and fill them adequately
- Wrap the stuffed leaves with another large leaf tightly
- Press down the stuffing in a 1-gallon jar, removing air bubbles from the jar - let it sit for at least four days
- Kimchi is ready - sprinkle sesame seeds and enjoy

Sauerkraut

Organic sauerkraut is a flavorful food that helps use easily add some good probiotics to our diet, and is easy to make at home with this simple recipe.

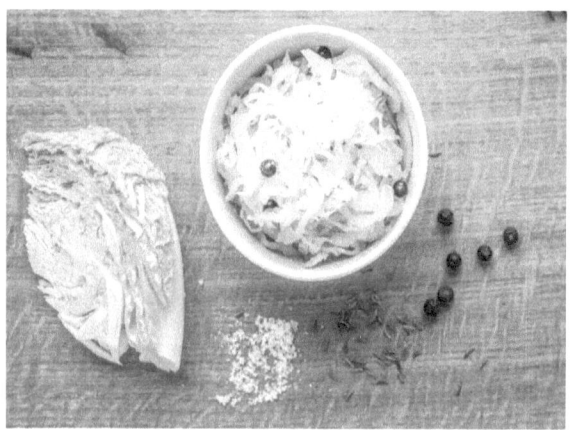

Ingredients
- 1 Head of Cabbage
- 1-4 tbsp sea salt

Directions
- Chop cabbage and sprinkle with salt
- Knead the pieces of cabbage or use a potato masher to mash them until they release liquid
- Stuff the mixture into a quart jar by pressing it underneath its liquid

- Use a tight lid to cover the jar
- Let it culture at 60-70°F for 2 weeks - once you get the desired flavor, burp the container daily to release pressure
- Sauerkraut is ready - cover the jar with a tight lid
- Move it to cold storage to develop more flavor

Lacto – Fermented Salsa

Lacto - Fermentation stimulates bacteria or microbes to produce lactic acid. It helps preserve vegetables and converts them into healthy probiotics.

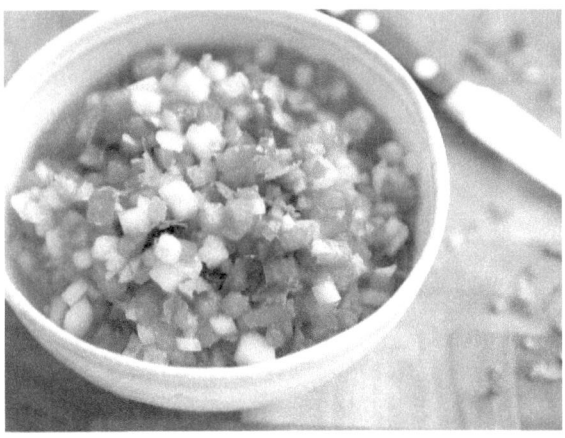

Ingredients
- 1 onion (diced)
- 2-3 large tomatoes (diced)
- 1 green pepper (diced)
- 1-4 jalepeños (diced)
- Garlic cloves (minced)
- Fresh cilantro
- Lime juice
- 2 tsp. salt or kefir

Directions
- Mix all the prepared vegetables, including whey, salt, or kefir
- Place the mixture into a fermentation container, and press down to release liquid - try to submerge vegetables under the liquid
- Add some extra water (if required)
- Let it ferment for 2 to 3 days at 78 degrees Fahrenheit
- Once fermentation is complete, store salsa in the refrigerator

Tempeh

Tempeh is a staple protein, and it is native to Indonesia. You have quite a few ways to cook it and can be prepared and used in a few different styles and can be served with meatballs and vegetables. You can cook it with meatballs and vegetables. The delicious protein and probiotic-rich recipe taste best with Teriyaki sauce.

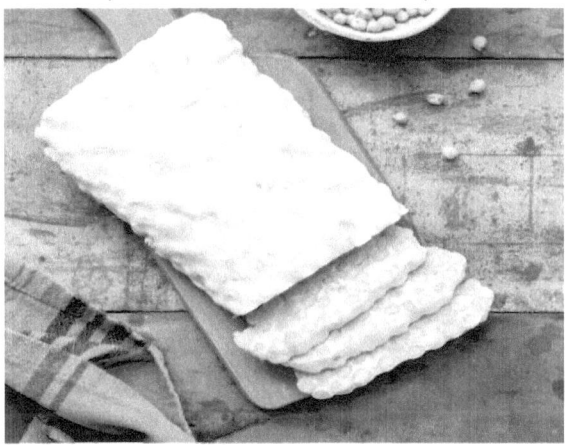

- 1 8 oz organic tempeh (cubed)
- 1 tbsp olive oil

Tempeh Marinade
- 3 tbsp veggie broth
- 1 tbsp tamari
- ¼ tbsp garlic powder
- ½ tbsp onion powder

Teriyaki Sauce
- 4 tbsp tamari
- 1 tsp olive oil

- 2 tbsp maple syrup
- 1 tsp hot sauce
- 1 tsp apple cider vinegar
- 1/2 tbsp garlic powder
- 1/2 tbsp corn starch

Directions

- Steam square-shaped tempeh for 10 minutes and mix all the ingredients and gently whisk together
- Place tempeh in a pot and pour marinade - marinate it for 15 minutes
- Sautee marinated tempeh in olive oil until crispy
- Mix all the ingredients of teriyaki sauce and add tempeh
- Heat the sauce to caramelize it and leave it for 3 minutes to thicken

Miso

The popular fermented food is widely eaten in Japan and is an essential part of traditional Japanese cuisine. Like other fermented foods, you can cook miso in a variety of ways. We have added a recipe of Garlic Miso-Glazed Salmon here.

Ingredients

- 500 g salmon
- 3 garlic cloves
- 1 ¼ tbsp fresh ginger
- 1 tbsp miso pasta (A traditional Japanese seasoning produced by fermented soyabeans)
- 6 tbsp honey
- 2 tbsp soy sauce

Directions

- Combine honey, soy sauce, garlic, and miso pasta in a bowl and mix well
- Mix marinade and fish and refrigerate them for 30 minutes for marinating
- Sear Salmon in a hot pan for one minute
- Once cooked from both sides, transfer it on an aluminum foil and bake it at 180 degrees Celsius
- Serve the crispy and glazed miso salmon

Beet Kvass

Sour, salty, and earthy - this jewel-toned beverage is Lacto-fermented and rich in probiotics goodness. The drink can be brewed easily and affordably. The preparation process is not much different than making sauerkraut.

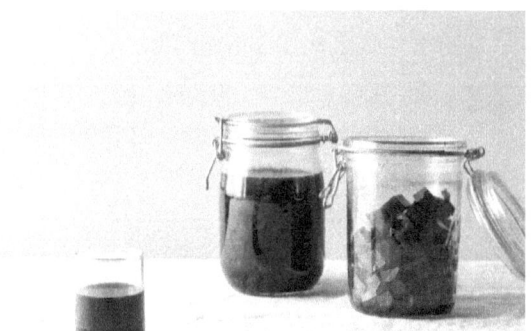

Ingredients

- 13-ounce beets
- 1 to 2 tsp Kosher salt
- Optional flavorings, such as lemon and spices

Directions

- Scrub and clean the beets and dice them in precise size and shape
- Place them in a jar and add salt with other flavorings and spices
- Add water and leave 1-inch headspace in the jar
- Let the beets ferment at room temperature

- Taste the beverage and release gases during fermentation
- Strain and store Kvass in the fridge

Chapter 6: The Role Of Probiotics In The Future

The Current Stance Of Probiotics In The Human Health

The new molecular techniques and clinical trials, ranging from studying probiotics to identifying new intestinal microbiota, have provided new perspectives about probiotics. The abundance, diversity, and dynamics of the gut ecosystem are still in the revolutionary phase. The current studies are proving the optimal impact of microorganisms on their hosts.

Most of the research on gut microbes has its focus on the evaluation methods of Gastro Intestinal Tract (GIT) bacteria's survival and their functions, plus the interaction between probiotics with a human's immune system has become one of the main subjects of studies. Numerous clinical studies have generated data to reinforce the powerful effects of microbiota or probiotics on human health.

A substantial number of studies support the idea that daily consumption of probiotics affects human health in many ways. The studies have demonstrated the mechanism gut microorganisms use to survive in the GI tract. Moreover, the demonstration also includes the way probiotics interact with already-present microbiota. The results show that both probiotic interaction and mechanism can have effects on the physiological functions of the host.

Thus, the effects of gut microbiota have received a lot of attention from the researchers. Many companies have commercially explored the way probiotics can benefit human health.

Can Probiotics Prove To Be Revolutionary For Human Health In The Coming Times?

Nonpathogenic microorganisms and probiotics confer many health benefits if administered in optimum amounts. Probiotics not only prevent, but may also alleviate the symptoms of some chronic diseases. They are the natural and temporary constituents of intestinal microflora.

In modern times our diets are becoming more and more processed, less raw, and more genetically modified which has led to the need for supplementation and the consideration to add a variety of different probiotic rich foods into our diets. The right concentration is essential for the human immune system, intestinal epithelium, and microbiota to promote an overall health. These components are vital for the maturity and proper functioning of your GI tract. Using immuno-suppressive therapy, antibiotics, and radiation may alter the composition of gut bacteria and can affect gastrointestinal flora.

Therefore, the incorporation of beneficial bacteria in your daily diet is an attractive solution to re-establish and revive the healthy gut microbiome. That means the efficacy of probiotics in acute post-antibiotic syndromes and enteric infections is evident now. There is growing evidence for an active and optimal role of probiotics in a wide variety of health conditions such as IBS, Colitis, Crohn's disease, Obesity, and much more.

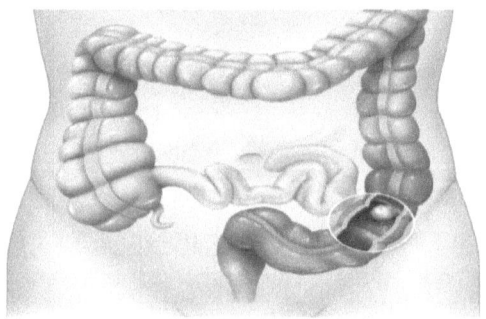

Conclusion

It is evident that the addition of quality, diverse Probiotics and Prebiotics into our daily lifestyle will impart so many varied health benefits. Their ease and safety of use, combined with their effectiveness and accessibility in either supplement or in dietary form, should make them an integral part of our diets. Not only for those suffering from different diseases, but for people who want to support and strengthen their gut microbiome to reduce risk and improve overall health.

Probiotics & Prebiotics support the gut and a happy gut microbiome supports us, and keeps many systems of our bodies, happy, safe & healthy.

Appendix

Probiotic Supplements

BlueBioitics Ultimate Care
The supplement is one of the top picks when it comes to choosing the best probiotic strain. BlueBiotics supplement contains 61 billion live microbes per serving. It contains S. Boulardi, which is an expansive and effective probiotic strain. The small capsules are specially formulated to resist gastric acids as they contain the highest living cultures.

Flora Critical Care
This supplement has the top ten strains with billions of probiotics per serving. They are vegetarian capsules, free of any potentially hazardous fillers, and binders. Ultimate flora contains a high number of general probiotic bacterial blends.

Garden Of Life Raw Probiotics
The supplement includes 13 strains of probiotics, including Bifidobacterium and lactobacillus. It also has two powerful variants of bacterium Streptococcus thermophilus. The supplements come with enteric-coating that keeps supplements safe from degrading under

the action of gastric juices before they reach the intestinal tract.